Encouraging Principles

Encouraging Principles

A PRACTICAL GUIDE TO POSITIVE THOUGHTS AND INSPIRATION FOR HEALTHCARE WORKERS

Diane Campbell

authorHOUSE®

AuthorHouse™ UK Ltd.
1663 Liberty Drive
Bloomington, IN 47403 USA
www.authorhouse.co.uk
Phone: 0800.197.4150

Published by AuthorHouse   10/07/2013

ISBN: 978-1-4817-6877-1 (sc)
ISBN: 978-1-4817-6878-8 (e)

CONTENTS

Dedications

This book is dedicated to all nurses, my mentors, colleagues, and others in the medical field that I have worked with, and finally, to all who have supported me throughout the years. I thank all the powerful women who have crossed my path. Firstly, I thank you, Lillian, my biological mother, for teaching me about principles when I was a child. Now that I am a grown woman, those principles remain. Thank you also for your constant prayers and support. Love you, Mummy.

Next, I dedicate this book to my spiritual mother, Joanne Morgan, whom I love so much. Thank you for the unconditional love and support you have given me. Your words, "You can do it!" are my favorite, and you are a rock, not only to me but to others. You are a wonderful person and a true mother.

I also dedicate this book to another mother and mentor, Veronica Pitt. You are my best friend, and words cannot describe all the kindness you have shown me. You are my counselor; you have helped me make decisions in difficult times. Thank you for your honesty and love. It made me who I am. You are a special person who has always shown commitment, compassion, and care to everyone. When you want to get the best out of me, your favorite words are, "What is this?" I had to shake myself up quickly "or else". You bring out the best in me. Thank you.

Finally, I dedicate this book to the rest of family and friends. I love you all.

—Diane Campbell

Preface

Communication has a set of tools that all health care professionals should have. Think of it as a "hat" that must be worn daily. In nursing, it is important to remember that each patient is unique; thus, it is important to use communication in different ways. Always remember "the how", "the when", and "the why" of what you are trying to accomplish and think about the consequences and the impact that your communication style has upon patients, their families, and your co-workers.

Communication is not just about words; it is a cornerstone in the expression of our humanity, and those who do it well can expect to benefit greatly. For example, positive attitudes, reassurance, support, confidence, commitment, and compassion are just some of the benefits, when one is an effective communicator. Compassion, for example, can be expressed through our body language when we are delivering individualised care to our patients. Working as a health care provider means there is an audience watching constantly. Therefore, as you walk "the hundreds of miles per day" to and from your patients, ensure that "grace" is with you in your words and actions. In this career, we have to deal with immense pressure. Staff shortages, low nurse-to-patient ratios, the huge paper burden (not just charting), learning new computer skills, and trying to keep up with clinical knowledge and new procedures are just a few things expected of nurses today. However, by being a team player, we can make a huge difference in all of the lives we touch: other nurses, doctors, patients, and families of patients.

In the health care system, the big "C" is not cancer but rather *communication*. Inappropriate or *mis*communication causes increased complaints and breaks down social interactions throughout NHS hospitals. Ideally, when we think of the NHS, we should think of compassion, care, commitment, smiles, good attitudes, efficiency, and respect.

Chapter 1

Lack of Communication and Motivation Increases Complaints

Langabeer (2008) defines a hospital as "an institution that provides medical and surgical treatment, where nursing care is provided for sick or injured people". During my career as a registered nurse with the National Health Service, I have encountered many sick and injured people. An NHS hospital is also a place where people should to feel safe to know that patient's health care needs will be met. Working for the NHS as a nurse is one of the most gratifying jobs anyone could have. It goes beyond providing patients with bed pans, writing up charts, and performing other routine duties. The most essential aspect of being a nurse is stepping into the role of the "communicator and motivator".

Communicating ongoing reassurance to patients helps them to make informed choices. According to Eric Hoffer, "What greater reassurance can the weak have than that they are like anyone else?" Further, when one is self-motivated, one can motivate others to ascertain their goals. For example, at work I would encourage student nurses to believe in themselves, to ask questions, and to work as a team. Moreover, facilitating communication can help improve health care worker motivation in many ways: better salary and job prospects as well as more positive relationships with co-workers. These things ultimately heighten patient satisfaction. Brian Tracy (2008), cited in Wilson (2009) said that "if you wish to achieve worthwhile things in your personal and career life, you must become a worthwhile person in your own self-development." Through self-development and having a more integrated, positive working environment, the nurse's focus naturally shifts to the patient's experience, which ultimately leads to better patient care.

It is always a frightening experience when a patient is admitted to a hospital for the first time. The nurse's role is to empathise with the patient and to anticipate his or her needs. A patient who is crying or feeling anxious may not necessarily be in physical pain. However, often the patient *says that they are in pain*. Always remember that pain is what the person says it is and exists whenever he or she says it does, according to (McCaffery's 1968,) cited in (Mezey and Ivo Luc Abraham, 2003). In most cases the patient could be feeling rejected and hurt rather than pain. It is crucial to provide reassurance, and to support the patient as part of the "care process".

In the year 2013 there have being many controversies regarding the quality of care within NHS hospitals across the UK. The root cause highlighted in one report was a *lack communication and empathy*. In a 2010 *Daily Telegraph* article, Rebecca Smith stated that "nurses should be more caring and compassionate towards patients in order to restore public confidence in the NHS." She also mentioned that "although surveys show continuing high levels of satisfaction within the NHS, personal experiences of poor care are highlighted daily in the media." These "experiences of poor care" illustrate that many nurses are neglecting the fundamental principles of nursing and are thus neglecting their patients.

Another report by *The Mail* online (August 26, 2010) stated, "the number of NHS complaints soars to a record high of 100,000 in a single year. In addition, more than 40,000 complaints on hospital services have been related to 'all aspects of clinical treatment.'" These statistics paint a negative picture of the NHS, but clearly they do not take into account the sacrifices of those nurses who are committed to their work always provide excellent care. This same article printed the claim that "over 12,000 letters were written about the bad attitude of staff". Often health care workers who display a bad attitude are those who are not enthusiastic or motivated. For example, people who lack motivation and enthusiasm are most likely to be passive and blame their circumstances on others. Those who are motivated and enthusiastic are more energetic, positive, and always working on new goals to improve not only their own life but for better job satisfaction, which includes improving their attitude towards patient care.

Further, the article notes that 11,000 complaints were received about delays or cancellations to outpatient clinics. In an article by *The Daily Telegraph* (February 10, 2013), it is stated that 1,200 patients died needlessly between 2005 and 2008 due to the "systematic failure of the NHS in a central hospital". Further, the Department of Health released figures suggesting that over 3,000 patients could have died unnecessarily because of "failures" at another five NHS trusts. These tragic statistics are highlighting the careless behavior of our health care workers. I agree with Robert Francis, (2013) who says in his report that there are "failing at every level of the NHS and that the culture among Health care staff must change". Clearly, it is time to change our approach to health care, and to change the public's perception of how well health care workers are performing.

Chapter 2

Attributes of a Great Nurse

If it is time to change our approach, how do we accomplish this?

First, we must fully understand the relationship between *care* and *nursing*. Everyone has the ability to *care*, but *to nurse one must be trained*. Though nurses are trained to care, the statistics have shown us that many are not doing this well. Caring should be at the heart of every nurse. In fact, this is generally what draws people to the profession in the first place. Accurate *caring* involves developing the following attributes and skills: advocacy, compassion, commitment, empathy, competence, communication, and flexibility. With practice, these basic yet powerful attributes can become the second nature to anyone who is willing.

Advocacy

Advocacy is an important attribute that aids nurses to form positive relationships with their patients. An advocate is one who supports people who are vulnerable and are unable to care for themselves. David Dennison defines an advocate as "one who acts on someone's behalf or for another person". This involves giving the patient information and supporting them when decisions must be made. As an advocate, the nurse must ensure that the care environment is safe for the patient, while at the same time protecting them from further injury. Nurses also have a duty to protect the rights of the patient and to provide assistance when necessary. Without an advocate, patients who are unable to express themselves are in danger of losing their rights. For example, some patients may find it difficult to express their needs, especially if they are fearful or anxious.

In order to have a safe and strong recovery, a nurse must believe in his or her own ability to heal. Note that healing is not about praying for your patient, or telling them about a religion, it is about motivation. For example, motivating your patient to eat or to mobilise are ways of promoting healing. It is very important for a nurse to speak on their patients' behalf, to offer encouragement, and to reassure them. Patients often contend with emotional stress due to being in a hospital. Therefore, it is important to create a soothing, positive atmosphere by encouraging the patient to have confidence and trust in the person advocating on their behalf.

This does not mean one should "cross the line" and become the patient's "cheerleader". For example, a particular nurse could be a patient's favorite advocate on the ward, and this is where the advocacy must remain. Once the patient is discharged from the ward, the nurse should avoid further interaction with the patient, unless he or she is talking to members of the primary care team, such as the district nurses to arrange further continuation of care. The role of the district nurses is to visit patients in their own homes to dress their wounds and administer medication, whilst, providing support for the patients and their families. There are many nurses who advocate well, love what they do, do it with a fiery passion, and remain professional at all times. A true advocate goes beyond the call of duty. For example, while a patient is in hospital a nurse can assist a patient in, making a phone call home to ensure that their loves ones or simple the cat is okay or fed. Other patients might need financial help. A true advocate would speak to them about the situation and refer them to the correct care agency to acquire financial help.

Compassion

Compassion is caring and respecting those who are weak and suffering (Thompson, (2006). Compassion requires you to be empathetic, kind, patient, and concerned. Compassion differs from care in the sense that the key to providing *care* is to be alert and pay close attention to details, as one small mistake could result in putting patients' lives at risk. When accepting a position as a nurse, there are rules in place to protect you, the patient, and the hospital itself. These guidelines should be read carefully and clearly understood, and questions should be asked to clarify any areas of confusion before the contract is signed. Any breach of these rules could result in penal consequences.

Compassion, on the other hand, is a true love of helping people. Before contemplating becoming a nurse, one should examine their true sense of compassion, as this is the key requirement of becoming a great nurse. Sadly, *many* young adults are flocking to the nursing field solely because of monetary reward. Compassion is a powerful "tool" that is required by all nurses. A nurse should always express to the patient that he or she understands and feels desperately about their pain or confusion. A nurse should always develop a sense of awareness to create a positive care environment. For instance, an anxious patient who is going for an X-ray will benefit from someone expressing a warm and reassuring attitude towards them. This can be done by holding the patient hand, giving them a quiet, kind word, or providing them with a gentle smile.

Commitment

There is a code of conduct that all nurses must follow, and a nurse's job extends beyond his or her shift. For a nurse with pride, the moment the uniform is on, he or she is clothed in grace, dignity, and poise. Each time a nurse enters the workplace, you are performing a duty to society—a duty one should take great pride in.

A nurse cannot choose whom to build a relationship with. For example, a patient may request a particular nurse. If all nurses are truly committed to patients and their job, the patients will not praise just one nurse but will praise and look forward to dealing with everyone who works in that department. A nurse should be steadfast in the face of unclear circumstances. He or she should carries out ones duties fearlessly and with utter loyalty, cheerfulness, and dedication. A committed nurse is resolute.

Competency

There are no shortcuts in nursing. It simply isn't possible to "do the wrong thing" without someone noticing. Patients place their lives in the hands of nurses every day and trust completely that their nurse has the skill and desire to make them well. However, no matter how much a nurse thinks he or she knows, it is important to be humble and consider the advice of a co-worker or more senior nurse.

It is not possible to be competent if information required to execute the tasks properly has not been read and learned. Thus, regular reading to keep current is critical for all nurses. Read! Scientists are always researching, experimenting, and discovering cutting-edge technologies or drugs that could one day save someone. Keeping up to date with evidence based knowledge will expand a nurse's mind and enables her to think outside the box when difficult and irregular situations arise. A nurse should always be reading and learning something new. The completion of a degree is not the end of studying for a nurse. Keeping current by reading regularly is a key part of being a competent nurse.

Communication

Communication has nothing to do with gossip. In fact, it is quite the opposite. Communication brings clarity to a nurse's relationship with his or her colleagues and her patients. At the very least, a nurse is caring for another human being. Issues such as race, religion, and sexuality should never be factors when providing the best possible care. Further, a good nurse can always distinguish her feelings from her judgments. This skill may be the key to becoming a clear communicator. Because communication is such an important factor, I will explore it in greater detail later in this chapter.

Empathy

Empathy is the "power of understanding and entering into another person's feelings" (Riley, 2004). For a nurse, empathy truly is an art, as it must be balanced with effective communication with a patient who may be in pain or discomfort. For example, having empathy will enable a nurse to respond promptly to a patient who is in pain. A nurse with empathy should ensure that the call bell is well within reach of the patient. This small example may look insignificant but it shows how to demonstrate kindness and understanding and gives that patient a sense of security and feeling that their nurse truly cares. Good listening skills are also important, as it takes one's full attention to show empathy.

A good rule of thumb is to avoid talking over the patient. Instead, a nurse should put herself "in her patient's shoes". For example, when a nurse is maintaining a patient's personal hygiene, it is important that they talk to the patient about *them*, rather than about the nurse's own personal needs or issues. Sometimes, something as simple as offering a patient a magazine can make a world of difference in that patient's comfort. This is especially important to remember for those patients who will be away from home for an extended period.

Flexibility

Being prepared to work long hours, including overtime, is part of being a nurse. It is important to note that being tardy and disrespectful towards authority will not go over well with co-workers on the same ward and, by extension, the hospital. Because of the stress and long hours, maintaining a well-balanced lifestyle is very important for those in nursing. At times it will get overwhelming, and a good nurse always remembers that she is not alone. There are many others in exactly the same situation: perhaps someone wants to take vacation but cannot because they are needed as the hospital is short staff. Having a flexible "can-do" attitude can be the difference between encountering setbacks and difficulties versus being a successful nurse.

Putting all these skills and attributes together will result one to become a fantastic, efficient and competent nurse. Certainly, these will help him or her to gain a sense of confidence and have faith in one's own abilities. Further, a sense of patience will allow for better focus while on the job. Also, being helpful and empathetic to other nurses ultimately results in a much more positive work environment. It is unprofessional and unfair for a nurse to watch her fellow colleague bear the burden of administering care to a patient. While there are codes to follow and it may also be the personal wish of other nurses to work independently, a nurse who regularly asks if she can be of assistance is highly regarded. Even a simple act such as holding a chart while he or she executes a task can relieve a co-worker and make everyone feel part of a team.

A nurse needs to keep in mind that she is building a sense of integrity within, and being kind to others is a wonderful way to accomplish this. Kindness is one of the greatest legacies a nurse can leave behind.

Everyone has "bad days", and nurses often have many. Especially in a care environment such as a hospital, it is important to keep calm and approach the situation with humility. Patients can sense tension, so even if there has been a negative interaction with someone else, a nurse must always try to show the patient that he or she is calm and peaceful.

Regardless of emotions or feelings of disorganisation, a nurse should put her best foot forward and greet the patients with a smile. Even if you are seeing the twentieth patient for that day or for that shift. A nurse who treats her patients like royalty and with great respect will be rewarded. It takes a great deal of focus and practice, but this approach with patients and co-workers will help build solid relationships and an overall happier work environment.

Trust in the NHS needs to be rebuilt. The current lack of the big "C", communication, is a major contributor to some problem. Communication is a very effective skill that all health care workers must apply to their jobs. Communication goes both ways. Clearly, if patients, nurses, and their co-workers cannot understand one another, there will be problems and confusion. Further, being mindful of body language is important, as it can send a stronger message than written or oral communication. In other words, nurses must begin to change their approach to communication if they are having trouble at work.

Part of the key to doing this is having a positive attitude, especially regarding patients. Having a positive attitude will bring communication alive, which in turn fosters great teamwork. Teamwork is important because, especially in health care, everyone is working towards a common goal.

The consequences of inappropriate or "missed" communication are, first, endangering a patient's life and, second, causing issues with other health care professionals. It is important to have integrity and confidence when communicating. Speaking boldly and clearly enables others to understand *exactly what you are trying to say*. Further, proper communication in a health care setting will reduce the amount of complaints made by the patients and their families, because they are more aware of what is occurring around them.

If health care professionals do not communicate appropriately, patients' lives can be at risk. Some examples of poor communication include failing to hand over vital patient information to other colleagues, poor documentation and charting, and talking about personal issues during patient handover. These behaviors are unacceptable and could put patients' lives at risk.

Communication plays a vital role in securing co-operation and compliance while managing patients. Without solid communication, some care workers can fail in their duty of care. Communication in the work environment is such a huge issue that it should be improved upon daily. For example, hospitals are full of people of different languages, races, and cultures. Therefore, one needs to find out more about the patients, such as their likes and dislikes. One way of doing this is by engaging them in a dialogue, especially when measuring their vital signs or doing the hourly or intentional round. A nurse should always ask short questions, such as "Where are you from?" and "Who do you live with?" Also, asking them about their diet is important, to ensure that each patient is taken care of holistically. Something new can be learned from each patient if the time is taken to get to know them on an individual basis.

One should never make assumptions about people. For example, never assume that all patients eat meat. Such details should be carefully considered during admission of the patient to check the background information. Paying close attention to details is important, especially if the patient is unable to communicate themselves. In cases like this, get friends and family involved by asking them the necessary questions. Asking for more information is never a bad thing. Always consider "the who", "the why", and the "the how", and always think about the consequences and the impact your communication style has upon others.

He who has a "why" can endure any "how".
—Friedrich Nietzsche

CHAPTER 3

The Multicultural Care Environment

Within the health care setting, we meet and work with people of various nationalities and cultures. When working in a multicultural environment, it is important to respect an individual's age, ethnicity, disability, sexual orientation, religious beliefs, and moral status. To prevent disagreement, it is important to greet each person as an individual and to ask him or her how they would like to be addressed.

For example, I was born in the Caribbean and migrated to London as an adult. I have encountered several situations in which cultural differences made me uncomfortable. At my first place of work, I met an older gentleman. When I greeted him I said, "Hello, Mr Rox." He then asked not to refer to him as "Mr Rox." Instead, he would prefer I acknowledge him as "Rox." To me this was an odd request, and it put me out of my comfort zone. My experience of Caribbean culture had shaped my perception of how people should be addressed.

Many of my colleagues are from different countries in the world including English descent. Each country has its own cultural individuality. As we navigate our way through life, we will constantly encounter situations that shift our perceptions. It is important to tolerate cultural difference in order to create a peaceful care environment. Teamwork adds support to the individual first and to the team second. This helps to create a positive work atmosphere. It is essential to show respect for one another, and in a multicultural environment, it is important to note that each colleague and each patient has a different personality, including accents, languages, beliefs, and values. Cultural differences can sometimes make communication difficult. Zimmermann (2012) defines culture as a particular group of people that is influence by the same language, habits, social activity, and cuisine. Within the work environment there are different cultures. The result is often an atmosphere devoid of cultural understanding. Be mindful of words or phrases that convey different meanings. Some languages have specific words for concepts, whereas other languages use several words to represent a specific concept.

For example, I encountered a situation in which a person misunderstood the meaning of the word "ignorant". The individual was angry after being asked why she was getting "ignorant". She felt she was being referred to as "stupid". In the Caribbean, however, the word ignorant means "angry". In the UK, the official meaning of the word "ignorant" relates to a lack of knowledge, while in some places in the Caribbean (Jamaica), the unofficial meaning of "ignorant" is angry or quarrelsome. The latter is used quite commonly within the Afro-Caribbean cultural sphere and is acceptable when used in the correct context. In contrast, when this acceptable cultural practice takes place in the British culture it will pose a problem.

Understanding a culture and its people can be enhanced by knowledge knowing that culture's language. There are many words that are specific to the Caribbean or Creole dialects. For instance, in Jamaica, there is a cultural food delicacy known as "bulla". It is a baked sweet brown bun that is served with cheese or avocado. But do not make the mistake of asking a "Bajan" (Barbados) if they like it, as in their culture, the word "bulla" means homosexual (Crichlow, 2004). In summary, a nurse must always be cognisant of differences in culture, belief, and race.

If it is clear that there has been a miscommunication, often these differences can be the cause. The solution is to listen effectively, and, when in doubt, always ask for clarification.

CHAPTER 4

Communicating with a Positive Attitude

A practical and positive attitude will make your team successful. Effective listening is critical to gather or share information. Therefore, having the right attitude is important to foster productivity and excellence. It is important to have the right attitude when communicating, and it is a skill that should be cultivated by all care workers.

The importance of communication skills cannot be disputed. They are the key to enable a nurse to execute good judgment. Practicing these skills is also essential for improving performance and building character. Therefore, acquiring the right set of communication skills can improve an individual's overall attitude. While the actions of others cannot be controlled, we can certainly control our own. For example, building trusting relationships with colleagues and focusing on consistency enable a more positive attitude.

Language may present a barrier to effective communication. For instance, some colleagues may speak different languages in front of others. This can cause tension when others cannot understand what has being said. However, in most cases, nurses who speak the same language as the patient can easily interpret what patients are saying. If one speaks in a language that the receiver does not understand, then communication can fail. Therefore, it is important to develop your interpersonal skills by being more aware of the words you are using in front of colleagues and patients. Always seek feedback to ensure your message has been understood.

By exercising our interpersonal skills when challenging situations arise, we can prevent them from escalating. A nurse leader should be neither passive nor aggressive. Assertiveness is the key to understanding and respect. It aids in the ultimate creation of successful teamwork, and it earns us support.

There has been a lot of debate in the past few years regarding ethics in health professional environments. There are certainly grey areas, but recognising that your actions impact others is the first step towards ethical behavior. Two rules to follow when considering ethics:

- You should help others while respecting their dignity.
- You have a responsibility to others.

First, helping others while respecting their dignity is ethical. Riley states that being ethical is about commitment and positively valuing the wellbeing of individuals in society (Riley 2004). Every patient has the right to choose or refuse treatment, freedom of speech, and the right to be respected without being discriminated against. Therefore, nurses have a legal and ethical duty to value their patients' rights. For example, if a patient says he does not take sugar in his or her tea, that wish should be respected. It is important to know that we as human beings are different. We all have preferences, so respecting the rights of your patients should be paramount.

Second, remembering you are responsible for others is critical. One of the most fundamental responsibilities of a nurse is to ensure that the ward environment is safe for the patients. A safe environment is about surroundings and ensuring that all the equipment you need is safe to use. Removing clutter from the environment that might cause harm to your patients is another example of responsibility. Responsibility always stands side by side with accountability, which means that you are expected to demonstrate a minimum level of competence in your work environment. The nurse is responsible not only to his or herself but also for the patient as a whole. This includes their physical, mental, emotional, and spiritual health. No one exists in isolation, and while different cultures emphasise individual achievement, a nurse must co-operate with others on a daily basis.

This is *active listening*, a technique used in effective communication. By repeating back what was heard through paraphrasing, a nurse shows that she clearly heard what was being said to her. There are many advantages of using this technique. It affirms sincerity, as the person being spoken to can see that you really are listening. The reassurance of being listened to validates the other person as an important participant in the conversation. It also means that nothing gets taken for granted and that the other party is satisfied that they are being understood.

To conclude, we are a multicultural society and therefore must be mindful of what we say and how we say it. While this can be challenging, exercising good leadership and displaying positive management skills can make these situations easier to handle. Two key elements of communication are listening and respecting others. We can respect a person's individuality by having a positive attitude and by working successfully as part of the team. Effective listening to gather or share information is a critical part of communication. Finally, having the right attitude is the key to high productivity and excellence. It is also important to have the right attitude when communicating. It is a skill that should be cultivated by all nurses. By showing respect to someone, a nurse is showing how she herself would like to be treated. Leo Tolstoy and Anna Karenina said that "respect was invented to cover the empty place where love should be." Nurses should strive to value and respect their patients and colleagues.

CHAPTER 5

Moving Forward, Communication, and Change

The National Health Service (NHS) has long been criticised for its lack of efficiency. Huge government spending in certain areas and cuts in others have contributed to the problem. According to Denis Campbell and James Meikle in October 17, 2011, *Guardian*, the government's ambition is to save £20 billion in efficiency in England alone by the year 2015. Despite the £20 billion in savings, the NHS will only receive a 0.1% increase in its budget each year. According to Campbell and Meikle, "Hospitals are now bearing the burden of the NHS's £20bn efficiency drive" and "hundreds of patients died because of poor care."

Within this same report, those who regulate the NHS, the Care Quality Commission, said they have issued a formal warning to hospitals regarding the lack of properly qualified and trained nurses. It seems obvious that the £20 billion could be invested in staff training and used to increase the staff-to-patient ratio. This would result in better care and ultimately reduce complaints. Regardless, the best thing that health care professionals can do for patients is to change their attitudes and to deliver care in a better and more positive way.

Attention to care is falling behind and is being overshadowed by paperwork. Paperwork is very important, as incorrect data can result in terrible mistakes. Thankfully, there will be a transition to a highly computerised system, which should ease some of the burden. The pressure on nurses has been relentlessly increasing over the past few years. For example, nurses have been in charge of ten to fourteen patients during their shift. It is extremely difficult to care properly for that many patients at one time. A ratio of 3:1 or 4:1 is much more reasonable. It takes careful thought and planning to prioritise and provide proper care for even four patients! Often when problems arise, the nurse did not see it coming. It is often the little things that matter, such as not leaving the call bell within the patient's reach or forgetting to give a patient a drink of water. The parable of the boiling frog that (Senge, 1990) cited in (Jackson, 1997) spoke about describes such situations well:

> If you place a frog in a pot of boiling water, it will immediately try to scramble out. If you place the frog in cool water, the temperature will not scare him. The frog will stay put. However, if the pot sits on a fire, and the temperature is gradually increased, something interesting will happens. As the temperature rises from 70 to 80 degrees the frog will do nothing. In fact, he will show all the signs of enjoying himself. However, as the temperature increases, the frog will become weaker and weaker until it is unable to climb out of the pot. Although there is nothing restraining him, the frog will remain in the pot and boil to death. Why? Because the frog's internal apparatus for sensing threats to survival is geared to *sudden changes* in his environment, not to *slow and gradual* changes.

It is the same concept for a nurse when she is "thrown in the deep end"; she rarely knows where the challenge is coming from. This is especially true when a hospital is short staffed. Those nurses that truly care feel like it is a weight and want to ensure that all their patients get full attention. They strive to ensure that patients still receive the best care possible. It is always the small things that matter, such as being hydrated and fed, having a clean bed, and similar details. Without doing these things, patients will complain and health care workers will boil to death like that frog.

Feelings of incompetence and timidity are out of the question if action is required. This is especially difficult when one nurse has at ten to fourteen patients to care for at a time. The parable of the boiling frog can also be applied to this situation. To further illustrate my point, nurses in this situation can be too busy to communicate care in a positive way. Doctors often use medical jargon that patients are unable to make sense of. Some of these are (MI) myocardial infarction, (CVA) cerebrovascular accident (stroke), (COPD) chronic obstructive pulmonary disease, and (mane) tomorrow. Medical jargon that patients cannot understand causes a breakdown of communication, which causes complaints. Therefore, remember to take the time to break down complex medical terms into simple words that patients can understand. Patients are regularly submitting the same complaint: that health workers are too busy or distracted. It is like customer service: the customer comes first at all times. No exceptions. In general most people remember the bad things rather than the good, so try to keep in mind the following:

> *You are remembered for the rules you break.*
> —Douglas Macarthur

CHAPTER 6

Dealing with Vulnerable Patients

Another important consideration with respect to communication is when working with vulnerable people who have dementia. Patients with dementia have challenging issues that can be quite distressing, not only for the patients but for the family as well. As a health care worker it is vital to remember that these patients have a wide range of emotions and concerns. Their families will be very worried about their loved ones, and many will naturally experience emotions such as anger, grief, and shock. They have to adjust to this new reality and watch as their vulnerable family members undergo being in hospital, due to dementia or other chronic health condition. The more support they have, the better they will be able to cope. Some families will ask lots of questions while in hospital experiencing this for the first time, and it is very important to take time to answer them. This will make a world of difference. Remember that good communication is vital to ensure that the needs of patients with dementia are met. The families need reassurance and support.

A recent survey by Borland (2011) stated that "almost 12,000 patients found that staff were criticised for being rude, arrogant and lazy, too often refusing to treat their patients with dignity or compassion." Very few health care providers wish to work in an environment in which their colleagues are labelled as rude, arrogant, and lazy. There are several guidelines, such as the Code of Conduct, that support other local guidelines and emphasise that nurses should take full responsibility regarding how to identify and minimise anything that might harm patients. Despite various government guidelines and local policies, some nurses still forget to adjust their attitude, communication skills, and behaviour. As previously discussed, some of the reasons why some nurses show poor behaviour in the work place are that they are overworked or short staffed, they have little job satisfaction, or they may simply need an attitude adjustment.

By following some of these steps, nurse can feel fulfilled and satisfied in their job, while giving quality care to patients. Dennis and Wendy Mannering said, "Attitudes are contagious." Are yours worth catching?

Respect means regarding someone with high esteem. Therefore, respect yourself and you will be respected. Respect your manager and colleagues. Lateness to work is a sign of disrespect, as are signs of disinterest and resentment for other members of the team. Thus, keep in mind that the attitude and respect you show at handover will dictate what kind of care you will give throughout the day. For example, the nurse on the previous shift might have to stay longer to inform you about patients; another might rush through the handover and you might fail to hear something important. Therefore, always give yourself plenty of time to get to work, leaving plenty of time for the handover. Through this you will be able to ask as many questions as possible, this will improve care.

> A *true genius admits that he or*
> *she knows nothing.*
> —Albert Einstein

Always respect authority, those who are set over you. Work as if it were your last opportunity to impress not only yourself but the patient and your boss. Who knows? There may be a promotion around the corner. Always humble yourself. Being humble will distinguish the wise leader from the arrogant power seekers. Humility does not make you weak. Humility is a form of strength. It takes humility to ask questions. For example, consider a nurse with less experience, explaining or showing the more experienced nurse how to use a hoist (an aid to lift patients). The nurse with more experience could become defensive and not listen to the colleague's opinion. Otherwise the more experience nurse could be humble and realise that it is a good exercise for the less experienced nurse to show his or her understanding of using a piece of new equipment or preforming a clinical skill. It is good to allow newly qualified nurses to show off their evidence-based skills and training, as it will help to build their confidence. Humility will permit you to consider other people's opinions. If humility is present, it will allow growth, learning, and character building to take place. A humble person gives others a chance and seeks to learn what he or she does not know. Often, a less experienced nurse has new information to share.

Always remember that "no one is an island, no one stand alone." Each nurse's and each patient's happiness is paramount for a better NHS. We need each other. Humility is an important quality that all care workers should have within the work environment. It is about being courteous and respectful to others. Humility is the opposite of aggression and arrogance. It is a quality that allows us to meet the needs and demands of others, in any situation.

Humility dissipates anger and heals your inner man, in which this will send out a positive

*message to your patients that allows them to
feel that the atmosphere around them is fresh.
Humility allows us to see the dignity and
worth of all people. Reputations are destroyed
by malicious and spiteful gossip; consequently,
it is always nice to be sociable within the work
environment. When you hear the mouth of
gossipers open, refuse to get involved, walk
away and make yourself useful . . . If you are
humble nothing will touch you, neither praise,
nor disgrace, because you know what you are.*
—Mother Teresa

Don't act like a know-it-all. The answer you need
may be in your colleague's or patient's mouth. Even
if you know the best technique to get the job done,
do not make your colleagues feel inferior. Use your
knowledge in a positive, constructive, and assertive
way. If they are resistant, this may mean that you
have to find alternative ways of helping them.
Knowledge comes from experience, and the behavior
and attitude of care workers should be positive at all
times. Sometimes I have to develop mental toughness
to overcome my fears in difficult situation, such as
asking a question when I am not sure. For example,
I might have to ask my senior colleague to explain
to a distressed patient why their wound is taking so
long to heal. I would use words like, "So sorry to
bother you, but please can you help me explain to

this distressed patient why his or her wound is not healing quickly?" Even though I might have already explained and reassured the patient, I wanted the patient to be at peace. As a result, I would enlist in the help of my senior, who had more experience. Subsequently, this will make the patient feel better and safe. Paul J. Fleyer said, "Good work habits help develop an internal toughness and a self-confident attitude that will sustain you through every adversity and temporary discouragement." Therefore, I have learned that we cannot rely on ourselves when it comes to patient care. Having humility and admitting to yourself that you need help can bring positive results in a difficult situation.

CHAPTER 7

Honesty and Humour Make a Difference

Honesty is always telling the truth and being straightforward. Some powerful words from nursing school are good to keep in mind: sincerity, truthfulness, trustworthiness, honour, fairness, genuine, and loyalty with integrity. Remember, when expressing your feelings to your colleagues, always do it without sullenness. Do not exaggerate or overstate information, which can cause your colleagues to feel inferior. When it comes to patient care, it is not about *who is right*; it is about *what is right for your patients*. Instead of boasting about how good you are, help your colleague to achieve some of your knowledge that can be imparted in a positive way. Remember, we are all in the care environment for one purpose, and that is to deliver quality care and promote a better NHS. Always admit your mistakes and apologise to anyone that might be affected.

Honour your patients' beliefs, and be respectful of their nature and spiritual faith. Remember, providing privacy and helping a patient to have dignity are essential aspects of giving quality care. Always ask your patients how they would like to be treated, respect them, and give them personal space.

Try to ask yourself these questions each day:

- Did I do something positive for my patients?
- Did I make a difference in their lives today?

Daily, I reflect on the quote by Henry Moore, "What has this day brought me, and what have I given it?" Whatever issues a person may have, they are not bigger than the person. If something does not serve a nurse's purpose, he or she should decide not to take it on. A nurse has the ability to change his or her attitude towards the situation. If she laughs about a problem, it could change her perspective towards it. Finding humour in a situation reduces the chance that it will degrade into anger. Laughing is a celebration of "the good", and it can be a wonderful way to deal with "the bad". Laughing, like crying, is a way of eliminating toxins from the body. Since the mind and body are connected, laughter helps us to forget about judgements, criticisms, and fears. According to Mike Dolan, "Sometimes it is just enough to smile sincerely."

CHAPTER 8

How to Be Committed

Do you truly feel for the patients in your care? Would you do something totally different if given the chance? Commitment and hard work enhance job satisfaction.

Every nurse should ask themselves these questions:

- Are you a good team player? A good team player cares about his work. Be reliable, respect others in your team, and communicate positively and productively.
- Have you got enough resources to get the job done? Having enough resources will increase efficiency and help you spend quality time with your patients.

- Is your work environment cluttered? Take the initiative to ensure that the ward environment is clean and tidy. A cluttered environment will affect your behaviour. For example, too much clutter around the nursing station could frustrate you when you are looking for patients notes. The NHS has put in place the Institute for Innovation and Improvement model, "the productive ward", to organise your work environment in a structured way. By following this model, your environment will be safer and your patient will have a better care experience.

- Do you feel stress at work? If so, find time to de-stress. A positive way to de-stress is to identify your excuses, habits, and attitudes. Stress begins in the mind, and according to and Nally and Bliss (2000), stress introduces thought and feeling. A positive thought brings about positive feelings. The essence of your contentment comes from the love and the relationship you have with yourself.

- Is your work environment always short of staff? Staff shortage is a major issue in the NHS. In *The Telegraph* (January 19, 2013), Laura Donnelly and Alison Moore stated that "hospitals pay out £1,800 a day for a nurse in NHS crisis." People's lives are priceless. Thus, it is important to let those in management know when there is a problem. When there are shortages, the nurse has a number of ways to complain:

- Use the incident form
- Ask other wards that are fully staff
  ○ Talk to immediate managers
  ○ Talk to the site managers

When doing this, remember that "a smile can brighten the darkest day."

—Mother Theresa.

CHAPTER 9

The Hope of Every Patient

Encouraging facial expressions will help patients to be more relaxed, thus enabling them to communicate more. The beauty of a smiling face will radiate light, good energy, and healing. A smiling face shows that a nurse is happy and she cares. Patients will feel this energy. A happy face promotes healing in patients and prevents long hospital stays. In my own experience of communicating in the work environment, a good communicator does not need to shout or need to be loud. A good communicator listens, shows warmth, and uses the right gestures to show that she cares, not only for the patient but for her colleagues.

I remember approaching a patient in his late sixties to take his vital signs. After introducing myself to him, he gave me his consent. I took his blood pressure, which was 122/70. He told me that I have a calming effect on him, as his blood pressure used to be within the range of 150 to 160. I was flattered, as I was not aware of any particular actions with him. I was just doing my job, and it was nice to know that I made the patient feel secure. The patient also told me, "If the nurse is not calm, it can be frightening. Lying in the hospital bed with someone standing over me is an awful experience." He continued to tell me that at the end of any procedure a nurse performs, he prays that he is going to be all right. I believe that this statement is the hope for every patient; they just want reassurance that they are going to be all right.

Remember that communicating well with your patients not only eliminates complaints, but it also provides better care, prevents abuse, and enhances healing for the patients. Not communicating with patients is a form of neglect. Don't forget that communication is the key to good nursing care. It is essential that nurses remember the different types of communication styles and utilise them in a suitable manner in the work environment.

Here are some quotes of encouragement from Mother Teresa to keep in mind while working:

- "Every time you smile at someone, it is an action of love, a gift to that person, a beautiful thing."

- "Let no one ever come to you without leaving better and happier. Be the living expression of God's kindness: kindness in your face, kindness in your eyes, and kindness in your smile."

A nurse's tone of voice will give patients confidence and let them know that they are in safe hands. Listening actively will prevent mistakes and reduce complaints. As nursing is a twenty-four-hour job, do not hurry. Take time to listen. Touching them and treating them with empathy will help your patients to trust you. Nurses, you are licensed to touch, so do not be afraid to touch or shake the hands of your patients. This will convey your good intentions. However, remember to ask their consent first. This shows that you respect their culture, privacy, and dignity. Even if you are not experienced or competent in that area of work, patients will tell you that you are the best nurse they have ever met, which is encouraging. The way a nurse appears is also a form of communication: a spotless uniform, neat hairstyle, and polished shoes will convey that you are neat and orderly. This will send positive energy to the patients.

Excellent posture is also important. Inappropriate body posture will not only send a negative message to the patients but will also cause your colleagues to wonder what they have done to upset you. This is not something nurses should have to worry about while on shift, as the patients care should always be top priority. Patients can receive a negative first impression of you when your body language is inappropriate. It is important to know that behaviour and moods change daily, but the key point is to be consistent in your perceptions and your own ability to handle events. At the point of beginning care, always introduce yourself to the patient, gain informed consent, and tell them what you are going to do. Maintaining confidentiality is a significant aspect of care. The Code of Conduct sets rule for us to follow. A nurse must respect a patient's right to confidentiality. Confidentiality is a fundamental aspect of human rights and must be respected at all times.

A nurse should talk to her patients and find out their likes and dislikes. Knowing their likes and dislikes and respecting these will help the patient to feel relaxed. For example, a patient who just had heart surgery may like to sleep in the chair rather than on the bed. It may not look ideal, but it is what is comfortable for the patient that matters. Nurses need to develop their own approach and become a therapist for their patients. Most patients just need someone to talk to. Sometimes a patient can end up in hospital unplanned. As their nurse, you must find out these details, as the patient needs reassurance to reduce their fears. A lovely message of reassurance from Pope Theodoros the Second is that "even if humans feel lots of fear, remember God will take care of you." This message is very important, as fear can be contagious.

CHAPTER 10

Your Behaviour Shapes Your Environment

Always ensure that the patient's environment is safe, especially if your patients are older people, if they have had surgery, or if they are vulnerable in some other way. It is important to know that when the patient lies in that hospital bed, they are vulnerable. Most patients are not used to hospital beds, and lying in them makes them feel insecure. Remember almost all patients feel vulnerable; they are at the mercy of their caregiver's hand. Therefore, respect and a shower of love goes a long way. Never forget to give patients plenty of water of drink. If the patient cannot use their hands, help them, as water saves life and prevents low blood pressure. Water helps the kidney to remove impurities from the blood, increases urine output, and helps prevent infection. Remember, a good shower of urine is the first line of defence against bacteria.

Once the patient is drinking, it increases the likelihood of bedwetting. Never leave a patient in a wet bed. If the patients in your care are older people with dementia and is within the age group of eighty to ninety years old. They may have problem in controlling their bladder and in most cases, they may have lost the elasticity in their bladder that control the urine. Also, due to their dementia, and memory loss, they may wet their bed. Therefore, these patients will have to wear incontinent pads, and will need an enormous amount of support in this area.

As mentioned before an older person may also have lost their memory due to dementia. Dementia can affect a part of the brain that enables a person to lost touch with the world around them. A person with dementia subsequently could lose their insights about everything, that used to be normal to them. It is easy to take these things for granted. For example, a patient with dementia will urinate and have a bowel movement but may not be aware of doing so. It is the nurse's responsibility to ensure that while these patients are in your care; their dignity is maintained to the highest standard. As they have no control over this situation, they depend solely on their nurse for help. These people cannot always give consent.

However, still, it is important to always explain to them what you are going to do. Changing their bedding and clothing immediately, is vital, as being in a wet bed will cause additional health problems, such as pressure sores and infections.

Nurses will often say, "I am going for my one-hour break now" after working four to six hours. A break is important, but waiting so long to take one can be exhausting. Instead, take small breaks as often as possible to keep a level head. Frequent "time outs", such as having a cup of tea or water, are essential. Statements like "I'm tired!" are not conducive to a healthy work environment.

Never be afraid to ask the patient's family to help. They normally love to help. Enlist the family's help in filling out forms, especially upon admission. Obtaining the pertinent details of your patients, especially the elderly, can be difficult when memory is a problem. Also, when families come to visit, have them help with feeding or with encouraging their loved ones to drink. It is nice to involve them, and they are generally pleased to help. Always offer cups of tea or coffee to the relatives. Telling them that the tea and coffee is only for the patients can be quite offensive. A warm beverage can go a long way in soothing fears and anxieties. Always view yourself as working for the most special people you have ever met. This is a powerful tool and the reward is limitless. Remember that it is not *what* you do that counts; it is *how* you do it. Your environment shapes your behaviour, and your behaviour shapes your environment.

Keep the ward environment as noise free as possible. Do not bang doors and bins. Try to dispose of boxes quietly; crushing them with your legs can cause added noise for your patients. Avoid speaking loudly, especially at night. Night is a time for people to sleep, and trying to sleep in an unknown environment can be quite stressful. A good rule of thumb is to pretend you have a headache. This will make it easier to move quietly and reduce the amount of noise pollution for the patients. When people are admitted to hospital, it is their "home" for the length of their stay. Thus, receiving their treatment in a quiet, stress-free environment is of the utmost importance. Patients are out of their comfort zone in hospital, so try to keep the noise level down.

Try to perform your job with pleasure and take pride in achieving goals. Every nurse should ensure that her job is being done with excellency in mind. A colleague once said to me that I "wears my heart on my sleeve" when caring for the patients. I was surprised to hear this, because I thought that when you care in any circumstances, you care with your heart. I then told my colleague that I did not become a nurse just to wear the name *nurse*. I became a nurse because after loving Jesus Christ, caring for people is my greatest passion in life.

Put on a positive attitude, and remember what you wrote on your curriculum vitae. Anticipate patient needs and never allow them to suffer in silence. Recall the words you must have used in your job interview: committed, compassionate, hardworking, team player, and motivator. Do not be deceived by inappropriate behaviour, as it will be found and dealt with. Carry on and be strong. Always assess yourself daily by keeping a log book of your strengths and weaknesses. Work on your weakness and extend your strength to others, such as student nurses, and you will be amazed by how skilled you will become in your place of work.

Chapter 11

Awareness of Actions

Love and work are the cornerstones of our humanness.
—Sigmund Freud

In my opinion, self-assessment and self-awareness are two of the finest tools for enabling solid communication within a work setting. Self-assessment requires health care professionals to gain insight into current evidence-based practice. Subsequently, it enhances the ability to recognise strengths and weaknesses. Self-awareness is the concept of acknowledging what is right and wrong and doing the right thing. If a nurse is able to evaluate her own mistakes, she can be more empathic to others. Self-awareness will help a nurse to use current evidence-based knowledge therapeutically and in leadership activities. It can increase the ability to both listening to others and to communicate. Constructive feedback from others will benefit health care workers by improving their communication skills, which facilitates better professional relationships. Through self-awareness, communication will become easier, as it allows health care workers to be assertive while giving information.

According to Germer (2009), one important quality of self-awareness is compassion. Compassion helps nurses to demonstrate patience and kindness. One way of showing compassion is to reward patients. This can be done by communicating care with honesty and integrity, which can be heartfelt when one is true to themselves. As Oprah Winfrey says, "Truth allows you to live with integrity. Everything you do and say shows the world who you really are. Let it be the truth."

Knowing what motivates and affects ones behavior will enable a nurse to be trustworthy by influencing others in a more collaborative and respectful way. It is therefore important to invest quality time in a personal development plan and take time to reflect upon it daily. Remember to allow love to show through in all actions and behaviours within the workplace. A nurse who allows her love for her job to radiate to each patient will reap rewards. Do not depend only on words to show love. Words must be supported by behaviour. Love is not impatient. Impatience can cause irritated reactions towards others and raise stress levels. It causes frustration and is a sign of dissatisfaction. Some people can become impatient due to hunger, dehydration, or tiredness. Once a nurse has identified the things that make her feel impatient, she can guard against them and prepare herself to face them and avoid negative reactions.

Health care workers should always speak to patients in the way that they themselves would like to be spoken to. Patients come first, and the reward is their healthy recovery after they have received the best treatment possible. Mario Andretti says that "desire is the key to motivation, but it is determination and commitment to an unrelenting pursuit of your goal—commitments to excellence—that will enable you to attain the success you seek." A professional relationship must be kept at all times, by identifying boundaries. Limits and behaviours can be defined in a nurse-patient relationship. For example, some patients prefer to be cared for by a male nurse; that is a boundary. The limitation is that the patient does not want a female nurse to be involved in their care. Respect the patient's wishes, communicate them clearly during handover to your colleagues, and maintain these boundaries.

Generally speaking, setting boundaries is about maintaining a positive relationship. Unhealthy relationships always lead to inappropriate communication and complaint. Therefore, it is our responsibility to maintain a healthy relationship with our patients and colleagues.

CHAPTER 12

Patient Expectations —Breaking Bad News

It is human nature to expect the best out of life; this is more evident when you are a patient. However, there are those who will seek attention and "play" the sick role. The "sick role", described by Talcott Parsons in the 1950s and cited by Sheaff (2005) is the social behaviour displayed by people who are sick and the people around them. An example might be a family member who is normally happy and cheerful. Suddenly they begin to sleep late, call in sick at work, and refuse to clean themselves. At first this behavior might frustrate and anger his or her loved ones. However, this might change if the family member goes to the doctor and is now diagnosed with depression. The doctor could commence this person on "sertraline", a medication that used to treat people with depression. Sertraline may cause serious side effects, such as high fever, sweating, and confusion.

On the other hand, there are patients who are not sick but will seek treatment for something. For example, when I was student, there was a patient admitted to the ward claiming that she was in pain. She was given intravenous fluid (IV) and analgesics for treatment. The doctors could not find anything wrong with this patient. After thirty minutes, doctors asked the nurses to stop all treatment for this patient. They found, after reading the patient's history that she had travelled from one hospital to another claiming that she was sick.

In every profession there are expectations and standards to adhere to. Within the health care profession, the Nursing and Midwifery Council (NMC) sets out a code of conduct that is imperative for nurses to follow. All health care workers are accountable and responsible for the patient and the duties that they perform. The (NMC) has set good standards in their code of conduct for nurses to follow. Nurses owe patients a duty of care. They are required to document every action performed on the patient, daily.

Nurses support doctors while breaking bad news to patients. Breaking bad news can cause psychological trauma, not only for patients but for their families as well. For example, a nurse may stand with the doctor to offer reassurance and support to the patient. Handling bad news differs from patient to patient. For example, as a student nurse I was asked to support and offer reassurance to a woman of Caucasian origin whose husband had just died. As I approached her, offering her a cup of tea, with tears filled my eyes. Suddenly! She was cursing her dead husband saying, "Just like him to bloody die on a bank holiday weekend. This means I won't be able to sort the funeral out until Tuesday. Just like him, to bloody die!" Another time, a child was brought into the Accident and Emergency department (A&E) having died of cot death. The parents were of African-Caribbean origin and were beating the floor, screaming, and rolling around on the floor wailing. They went to the extent of calling their pastor asking him to bring their baby back to life. They chanted prayers and blew breath into the child, whilst demanding the Pastor to raise the child from the dead as "Jesus did when He called Lazarus back to life". These two examples show how differently people can react to bad news and how reactions can depend upon culture.

All patients have a right to receive information about their condition, and it must be given with sensitivity, according to the patient's needs and respecting their wishes. The information provided should be accurate and truthful. In most cases the patient or their families are in fear and shock and need every ounce of reassurance they can get. For example, once a patient came to hospital, having pain in one of her leg and received the bad news that her leg would have to be amputated, due to ischemia. Ischemia means there is no blood supply to the leg. This kind of news can cause turmoil for the patient and family, especially if the patient provides the main source of income for the family. As a result, many lives will change, and the patient has to live with the emotional effects of losing part of her body, as well as perhaps being unable to cope financially. Helping patients to feel that they are not isolated or abandoned during difficult period is extremely important.

Another example is explaining to a patient that they have a urinary tract infection. This could cause the patient much distress if not communicated in a positive way. This should be done in privacy and with dignity. Reassurance is crucial, as the patient may feel the urinary infection could cost them their lives. Reassurance will help restore the patient's confidence, not only for themselves but also in their nurses. In this instance, a nurse must explain to the patient that this information will be conveyed to the doctor, who will prescribe the necessary appropriate treatment to combat the infection. Encouraging a patient with a urinary tract infection to drink plenty of fluids is important. This will help them to get over the infection.

When breaking bad news, it is important to keep communication style in mind. Ask open-ended questions and allow time and space for the patient to answer. Give the patient time to process the information and ask questions. Silence is golden; it is a sign that the patient has heard what was said and is trying to process it. At this point it is important not to rush, remembering to touch, have eye contact, and maintain a kind facial expression. This will give the patient support while allowing them privacy. Some patients can be fearful of expressing their emotions, hearing certain answers, or not knowing how to cope. Some may ask a lot of questions, while others may not know what to do. For example, a patient may ask, "How long will it take to better?" A nurse may not have all the answers, but this is an excellent opportunity to consult with the doctor. Some patients may even feel embarrassed about sensitive issues. In these instances, allow communication to come alive in each word. Think of the words as a "hat" and ensure that this communication hat is one of the finest hats ever worn by a health care professional.

CHAPTER 13

What to Expect as a Potential Qualified Nurse

For most patients and their families, being in hospital can be a worrying time. In many cases some patients do not have a family and have to face being in hospital alone. As a potential nurse, it is important to know that a patient can be admitted to hospital through many different routes, the most common route is the accident and emergency department (A&E).

In the A&E, you will find a lot of people who are waiting to be seen by a doctor or a nurse. Some of these people may be crying and in pain and are with anxious family members. It is important that nurses avoid feeling anxious themselves. There is always someone available to speak with who will help with relaxation. However, this is a good opportunity to practice some simple nursing skills, such as asking them if they are okay or showing them to the toilet. Also, if the patient is elderly, ensure they are lying in a dry bed or trolley.

Every patient in the A&E department will be seen by doctors, nurses, and sisters in the department. However, it is important to know that there are specific priorities in the A&E department. This department assesses and treats patients with serious injuries or illnesses, such as loss of consciousness, chest pain, breathing difficulties, severe bleeding, and other life-threatening health problems. If a patient has been waiting for two hours and another patient comes in with difficulty in breathing, chest pain, or other more serious issues, he or she will be seen first.

Nurses are always busy working hard to avoid long wait times for patients. Be conscious of the fact that patients get hungry; it is easy to offer them something to eat or drink. For example, a cup of tea. Be aware that not all patients waiting in A&E can eat or drink and can be nil by mouth (NBM) due to surgery. While some patients are unable to eat, ensure that they are hydrated. Always follow the protected meal time procedure. Anticipate their needs and never allow a patient to suffer in silence. Patients will have a lot of questions, so be prepared to answer them.

As a nurse, part of the communication process is assessing the activities of daily living (ADL) daily. This is a process in which the nurse draws any abnormalities from the patient. The ADL can help to assess whether the patient is sick or well. However, whenever someone is unwell, they must be assessed to find out what they can and cannot do, and what normal and abnormal behavior is for them.

As a potential nurse it is important to be familiar with the activities of daily living, according to Roper and Tierney (2002). There are twelve activities of daily living:

- **Breathing.** The air we breathe is important. Breathing is defined as taking in oxygen and expelling carbon dioxide. Unfortunately, some patients' breathing may be compromised if they have respiratory problems such asthma, emphysema, other lung diseases, or an obstruction affecting the respiratory airway or the lungs itself. A patient's respiratory rate can vary between 12 and 20 breaths per minute. One way of checking this is by counting their respiratory rate for one minute while watching the rising and falling of the chest.
- **Mobilising.** It is important to check whether the patient can mobilise, aided or unaided. It can be difficult for those who have had a major operation, such as heart surgery or a repaired

leg fracture. If a patient must remain in bed at all times, this can cause further complications such as chest infections, constipation, pressure sores, and stiff muscles. Also, If patient is not mobilising and is laying or sitting in the same position for a long time, the blood in the body will not be able to circulate freely, which may result in the risk of deep vein thrombosis (DVT). DVT is a clot formed in the leg and if bursts small clots of blood can travel to the lungs, causing further complications such as pulmonary embolism (PE). Shortness of breath is one way of identifying a pulmonary embolism. Thus, it is always important to know the level of mobility a patient has.

- **Controlling body temperature**. Normal body temperature can be 36.2 to 37.5 degrees celsius. Always check the patient's vital signs according to their condition. This means making sure that the patient is not hyperthermic (too hot), or hypothermic (too cold). A body temperature above 37.5 could be abnormal for the patient. Therefore, communicate this information to a mentor or the nurse in charge immediately so that action can be taken. To reduce temperature, paracetamol can be administered, clothing reduced, or, if the patient is not NBM, plenty of fluids given. On the other hand, during the cold months of winter, many patients can get chilled. Thus, it is important to ensure they have blankets and cups of tea to keep them warm.

- **Eliminating.** It is essential that a potential nurse encourages patients to communicate any abnormalities in their bowel habits. The pattern of their bowels is extremely important during an ADL assessment. For example, some patients can be constipated (have difficulties passing stool) or have diarrhoea (loose, watery stool). If a patient is constipated, it could be due to lack of fibre in their diet, inadequate hydration, or some other medical reason. If the patient has diarrhoea, first check the consistency then the duration of the movement. If it have been three or more days, the patient could be dehydrated, and this should be reported to the doctor immediately so that appropriate measures can be taken.

- Also, communicate with the patient to find out about their diet. A stool sample may be required to check for any microorganisms or bacteria. Refer to the nurse in charge regarding the hospital's infection control protocol. Ensure that your patient has lots to drink; they may want to use the toilet more frequently. Therefore, helping them to the toilet is important. Ways of doing this include giving them a bed pan, commode, changing their incontinent pad, directing them to the toilet or providing a urinal bottle. Also, encourage the patient to use to call bell and to ask for help.

- **Maintaining a safe environment.** This is essential for the patient's wellbeing. During assessment, speak with the patient about their safety needs. For example, are they wearing spectacles, ensure that there are no obstacles within reach of the patient. Check that their bed space is dry, the correct lighting is in place, and that they are wearing the correct footwear. These measures must be put in place to prevent your patient from falling.

- **Washing and dressing.** Identify whether the patient can wash and dress themselves. Find out from the patient or their family members how they manage at home. While the patient is in hospital, if they cannot wash and dress themselves, it is the nurse's duty to assist them in this area without taking away their dignity. Informed communication must be expressed. For example, always explained to the patient exactly what you are about to do, and be sure that informed consent is gain in every given area of care, if possible. Patients are vulnerable at this point so give them lots of reassurance, which helps them to understand that their nurse cares.

- **Eating and drinking.** Diet and fluids are important and are often neglected, especially for elderly patients. During assessment this area needs to be identified and addressed. Question the patient and family about their diet and fluid regime. If the patient is not eating and drinking properly, there may be need for extra nourishment and intravenous fluid. The patient may even need to be referred to the dietician for nutritional input. If a patient cannot feed themselves, the nurse must feed them. A food and fluid chart is important to document how much the patient has eaten at each meal time.

- **Expressing sexuality.** In assessment, expressing sexuality means understanding the patient's beliefs, attitude, culture, and spiritual mores. We are all sexual from birth, but it is not the nurse's job to question the patient's gender identity or sexual orientation. In these cases, it is important to show the patient that their body image and personal choices are respected.

- **Working and playing.** Try to find out the patient's social history, such as where they live and whether they still work or are retired. Check whether the patient lives alone and whether they are married or single. Also, find out the type of housing they have. This information will give you an idea about the type of home the patient comes from. Upon discharge, it is important to ensure that the patient will be returning to a safe home environment. There may be a need for an occupational therapist's assessment of the patient home prior to discharge.

- **Sleeping.** Some patients may find it difficult to sleep. Communicate with the patient to find out if there are any abnormalities in this area. Some patients may find it difficult to sleep in hospital due to a change in their environment. As a potential nurse, it is important to liaise with the nurse in charge, who will inform the doctor of the issues. Maybe, some patients take medication to help them sleep. Also noise can be a factor for hindering sleep.

- **Dying.** In dealing with potential death, it is important to find out the patient's and their families wishes. Some patients associate hospitals with death, so it is important to reassure them and try to alleviate any anxiety and fear regarding death.

As potential nurses, learning the activities of daily living will help you to understand the physical, social, emotional, and psychological aspects of patient needs. Never forget the importance of "the hourly round", as it is one way of communicating and getting to know your patients. In doing hourly rounds, patients will be able to communicate their needs and enable a nurse to act accordingly. A potential nurse may not be able to administer medicine independently. Thus use, care and diligent attention as a form of medicines to treat your patients.

Wherever, the art of medicines is love,
there is also a love of humanity.
—Hippocrates

CHAPTER 14

Days of the Week and Daily Routines in Hospital

For potential nurses, it is good to know what life is like on certain days in a hospital. Not every day is the same. Recognizing patterns will help you to feel more comfortable each day. Always know that each hospital's ward setting and care homes are different. This is the author's own perception.

Sunday

This can be the quietest day in the hospital. Doctors are called only for emergencies. There is less noise and fewer activities around patients. As there are fewer activities, there are fewer people around. On Sundays, families come to visit their loved ones. This is an excellent day to find out more about the patient, if they are willing.

Also, the patient condition must be taken into consideration. For example, some patients will require lots of attention. Always assess what communication style they prefer. There is a lot for you to work with, such as spoken words, touch, and eye contact (must be secure with good facial expression). As a nurse, your duty is to develop these general principles of communication with all patients. Take time out to sit with your patients and use other nonverbal approaches in communications, showing them warmth, respect, and sympathy. These are simple yet powerful skills that will take you through your career.

Monday

This day could be a crowded, busy day on any ward. Patients can find the hustle and bustle of Mondays to be overwhelming. For example, nurses must co-operate with consultants, registrars, house officers, first-year doctors, and medical students while examining a patient. It is best to explain to patients beforehand what each visit is for and what the expected procedure should be. Monday is assessment day, and many patients will have CT scans, chest X-rays, limb X-rays, and MRIs. NBM (nil by mouth) orders will be seen, and those patients would have had nothing to eat or drink for at least six hours. However, sometimes there is an order that a patient who is NBM can have water, black tea, or coffee. Normally, patients must stop drinking two hours prior to a surgical procedure. The reason for this is that anything in the patient's stomach is acidic, and if a patient has a full stomach during an operation, the food could move from the stomach to the esophagus, then into the breathing tube, which is the larynx causing aspiration or damage to the lungs.

Bloods can be taken from patients at any hour, anytime or any days of the week. However, often tiny amount of bloods are taken from patients on a Monday. This blood test is only to check if the patient condition is improving and for the Doctor to decide what treatment to give. For example, Potassium is an electrolyte that circulates in the blood of our bodies, use for the function of nerve muscles and cells, such as the heart. The normal level in the blood can range from 3.5-5.5 mmol, if a patient potassium level in the blood is above 5.5 mmol, the patient could be at risk of having a myocardial infraction (heart attack). Hence, bloods must be taken, to prevent any health risk. Also many patients will have a plastic tube called a cannula, inserted by a small needle into a vein on their arms. The needle is then taken away. The cannula can be left in the patient's arm for up to three days and this is a route to administer medication intravenously.

Tuesday

Usually patients are preparing for surgery on Tuesday. Many have had surgery. Doctors come to check on them. On this day, the nurse is the most important person to the patients. The pain nurse may come depending on the patient's pain level. The physiotherapist may come to introduce themselves and might help to mobilise the patients. This is to ensure that they are fit prior to going home. Encourage patients to eat. They may feel depressed and be internalising their sickness. This can cause a loss of appetite and delay their recovery.

As a potential nurse, take the initiative to encourage health promotion. For example, find out how many people in your ward or department smoke cigarettes. Also, you can look how smoking affects the body. This illustration will give you an idea how to promote health.

Matfin and Porth (2009) explain that smoking is a major risk factor that can be affected by a change in health care behaviour. Cigarette smoking is normally linked with cardiovascular disease, which can lead to death. For example, smoking over a long period can reduce blood flow in the body and cause the lining of the arteries to become hard and clog up with fatty material called atherosclerosis. Atherosclerosis can induce high blood pressure, heart attack, stroke, throat cancer, and diabetes mellitus (Matfin and Porth 2009).

Those of my friends who smoke claim that although it is habitual, it does relieve stress and anxiety, while some says, they smoke more when socialising. Others began smoking cigarettes from a very young age. Health promotion should be ongoing; however, when the opportunity arises and the family is around, this is a good time to promote health, as they can be involved. You could ask short questions such as

- How long have you smoked?
- How many cigarettes do you smoke a day?
- Do you eat less when you smoke?
- Would you like help to stop smoking?

You can develop a trusting relationship with your patient and use this strategy of communication to promote health. Firstly, give the patient a leaflet outlining the effects of smoking on the body. Secondly, if they are in agreement, the nurse can ask the doctor to prescribe nicotine patches. Thirdly, they can be referred to a smoking cessation team, who can follow them up. By following principles such as this, you can prolong your patients' lives, helping them to lead a healthy life.

Wednesday

Encourage the patients to rest. A good sleep helps them heal more quickly. They will likely not sleep well in hospital, but it is still important to encourage them to rest and get as much sleep as they can. A patient may not be sleeping well because they are in pain, anxious, worried, depressed, angry, or suffering some other emotional or spiritual problem. If the patients are in pain, do not hesitate to ensure that the appropriate pain relief medication is administered to them. Be sure to resolve any issues that will hinder them from sleeping. A carbohydrate snack is very helpful to aid in sleep.

Thursday

Anything can happen on this day. Patients may be going for scans or operations. This is the day that the patient could be admitted or could be going home. It is called an "unpredictable day" for this reason. Always have answers ready for patient's questions about their care. Ask the patient to write down the questions they want to ask (if possible). Sometimes the patient is suffering and refuses to let their voice be heard. It is important to know if the patient is to be discharged, whether from the accident and emergency department or from the ward. Thus, appropriate arrangements with the district nurses need to be made, if necessary. These nurses will go into patients' homes to dress their surgical wounds, leg ulcers and monitor their blood sugar if the patients are unable to. A discharge summary will be sent to their general practitioner. The discharge summary includes their length of stay the patient had in hospital and the details of any investigations and treatment they had during this time. In some cases a follow-up appointment is made for the patient to see their GP, or for a return visit to hospital, within six weeks. Upon discharge, the nurse and doctor will explain their recommendations for aftercare and reassure patients that if they face any abnormal problems they should not hesitate to come back to hospital, or to see their GP immediately.

Friday

The ward might be very busy. Every member of the team will be very busy with various commitments, such as discharges. For example, the physiotherapist will be making sure that patients are going home with the correct walking aid, if required. If the patient is elderly, the occupational therapist will ensures that the patient are going home to a safe environment.

As potential nurses do get involved, the key is to be motivated and ask questions. In general terms, motivation plays a vital part in your performance as a healthcare worker. If you are committed, you will be motivated and experience an increase in confidence. Indeed, motivation can play a vital role in your learning and development. A committed nurse will always acknowledge the need to develop and provide evidence-based care. Without professional development, your performance will not match the description of a "competent nurse". The Nursing and Midwifery Code of Conduct (2008) says a nurse must keep their knowledge up to date throughout their working life. Therefore, healthcare professionals should perfect their practice with standards of excellence.

Saturday

You will find that the ward is quiet; most people have gone home. It depends on the patient's condition, but some may still be trying to understand what brought them to hospital. The telephone will be ringing continuously at the nursing station, as most families are trying to get information about their loved ones. In most cases, the families are more anxious than the patients. However, reassure them and remind them that their family member is in safe hands.

Conclusion

Much of life is based upon communication, but it is especially necessary when people are in need of care. Learning to communicate well is an ongoing process. We all need each other and would otherwise have a lonely existence.

The NHS has evolved since the days of Florence Nightingale and Mary Seacole, who were the pioneers of nursing in their time. Then, it was strictly hands-on care. Now, however, we are caring for people on a different level. Today, the computer has taken over for much "paperwork". Further, nurses are required to have a degree rather than a diploma. Nurses are expected to become specialised and more autonomous, which is leading them to become true professionals and no longer seen as "the doctor's handmaid".

There are more policies, guidelines, and laws to adhere to. However, these policies are in place to enable health care providers to strive for excellence. Without them, the NHS would not be able to function. The purpose and role of a health care worker should be consistent and should ensure that "care" is the focus of our nursing career.

What we have done for ourselves dies with us; what we have done for others and the world remains immortal.
—Albert Pike

References

Bates, C. 2010. "Number of NHS Complaints Soars to Record High of 100,000 in a Single Year", *The Daily Mail* [Online]. Available at http://www.dailymail.co.uk/health/article-1305979/NHS-hospital-complaints-soar-record-100-000-year.html. Accessed January 8, 2013.

Borland, S. 2011. "Rude, Arrogant, Lazy: Patients" Verdict on NHS Staff as Two in Three Tell of Poor Care', *The Daily Mail* [Online] Available at: http://www.dailymail.co.uk/health/article-1359679/NHS-staff-rude-arrogant-lazy-Patients-verdict-2-3-tell-poor-care.html. Accessed May 20, 2013.

Crichlow, W. E. A. 2004. *Buller Men and Batty Bwoys: Hidden Men in Toronto and Halifax Black Communities*. Canada: National Library.

Francis, R. 2013. "The Mid Staffordshire NHS Foundation Trust Public Inquiry", Available online at: http://www.midstaffsinquiry.com/press release.html. Accessed May 27, 2013.

Germer, K. C. 2009. *The Mindful Path to Self-Compassion: Freeing Yourself from Destructive.* United States of America: Guilford.

Jackson, R. 1997. *Nutrition and Food Services for Integrated Health Care: A Handbook for Leaders.* United States of America: Aspen Publisher.

Langabeer, J., R. 2008. *Health Care Operations Management: A Quantitative Approach to Business and Logistics.* London: Jones & Bartlett Publisher.

Matfin, G., and C. M. Porth. 2009. *Pathophysiology: Concepts of Altered Health States,* 8th ed. Library of Congress: Lippincott, William, and Wilkins.

Mezey, M. D., and T. F. Ivo Luc Abraham. 2003. *Geriatric Nursing Protocols for Best Practice,* 2nd ed. United States: Springer Publishing.

Nally, B. E. and V. Bliss. 2000. *Recognising and Coping with Stress.* London: The National Autistic Society.

Nursing and Midwifery Council. 2008. *The Code: Standards of Conduct, Performance, and Ethics for Nurses and Midwifes.* London: NMC

Riley, B. J. 2004. *Communication in Nursing,* 5th ed. Missouri: Mosby Elsevier.

Roper, N., W. W. Logan, and J. A. Tienery. 2002. *The Elements of Nursing: A Model for Nursing Based on Model of Living,* 4th ed. London: Churchill Livingstone.

Schneider, R. H., MD, and J. Z. Fields, PhD. 2006. *Total Heart Health: How to Prevent and Reverse Heart Disease with the Maharishi Vedic Approach to Health.* United States of America: Library of Congress.

Sheaff, M. 2005. *Sociology and Health Care: An Introduction for Nurses, Midwives, and Allied Health Professionals*. London: McGraw-Hill International.

Smith. R. 2010. "Nurses Should Be More Caring to Restore Public Confidence: Report, 'Nurses Should Be More Caring and Compassionate towards Patients in Order to Restore Public Confidence in the NHS, a Government Review Has said'". *Telegraph UK* online. Available at http://www.telegraph.co.uk/health/healthnews/7351513/Nurses-should-be-more-caring-to-restore-public-confidence-report.html. Accessed May 10, 2013.

Thompson, E. I., M. K. Melia, M. K. Boyd, and D. Horsburgh. 2006. *Nursing Ethics*, 5th ed. London: Churchill Livingstone.

Wilson, K. 2009. *Hip Tranquil Chick: A Guide to Life on and Off the Yoga Mat*. United States: World Library.

Zimmermann, K. A. 2012. "What Is Culture? Definition of Culture," available online at http://www.livescience.com/21478-what-is-culture-definition-of-culture.html. Accessed May 27, 2013.

Recommended Reading

BBC News Health. 2010. "Record increase in NHS complaints Hospital: 'Written complaints about NHS hospital and community services in England has seen the biggest annual rise since records began over a decade ago'". August 25. Available online at http://www.bbc.co.uk/news/health-11083236. Accessed April 20, 2013.

Dominiczak. P. 2013. "Jeremy Hunt: Cut Red Tape to Prevent Another Stafford Hospital Scandal: 'Hospitals Should Face Fewer Inspections and Assessments in Order to Prevent a Repeat of the Mid Staffordshire Trust Scandal, Jeremy Hunt Has Said'", *Telegraph UK* online. February. Available at http://www.telegraph.co.uk/health/healthnews/9860639/Jeremy-Hunt-cut-red-tape-to-prevent-another-Stafford-hospital-scandal.html. Accessed April 20, 2013.

Donnelly, L. 2013. "Stafford Hospital: The Scandal That Shamed the NHS: 'Patients Lying Starving, Soiled, and in Pain. Over-Worked Staff Dogged by Targets. Laura Donnelly Tells How a Culture of Fear Meant That Ticking Boxes Trampled over the Basic Needs of the Most Vulnerable'", *Telegraph*

UK online. January 6. Available at http://www. telegraph.co.uk/health/heal-our-hospitals/ 9782562/Stafford-Hospital-the-scandal-that-shamed-the-NHS.html Accessed May 28, 2013.

The Authors Thoughts

I hope that you have enjoyed reading this book, and that it will help you in your place of work. If you are contemplating a career to become a nurse, a carer or still in nursing school, then use, the principles as a guide.

Hopefully, this book will be widely read, not only within the NHS, but by every, nurse working in Residential, nursing care homes, and internationally, in every area that people are being cared for.

The author hopes to visit each health care setting, to find out from colleagues if they have read this book, and how the principles benefit their practice. Ideally, the author would like to complete a survey to gather statistics on how many have read the book, have they implemented any changes , and whether the "principles" have made a difference to their lives and work environment.

This book does not end here! The author's ultimate goal is to one day see that her suggestions are making the world of health care a better place for all involved.

Lightning Source UK Ltd.
Milton Keynes UK
UKOW05f2139241113
221664UK00001B/14/P